Table of Contents

The Relationship Between Anxiety and Perfectionism: Understanding and Breaking the Feedback Loop

1. Introduction to Anxiety and Perfectionism

2. The Interplay Between Anxiety and Perfectionism

2.1. Anxiety as a Driver of Perfectionism

Perfectionism and Anxiety: How to Break the Cycle

1. Introduction to Perfectionism and Anxiety

Today, we've come to understand perfectionism not as healthy striving, but as "a personal predisposition rather than a learned trait." The fact that genetics contributes around 50% to perfectionism only adds to the hardwiring of this concept. So, from the word "go," a perfectionist is likely to be a highly anxious person—or just more anxiety-prone—so to say that perfectionism causes anxiety is not too far from the truth. Anxiety is one of the most common disorders worldwide, and it tends to co-occur with other disorders at a high rate. In this 10-part series, perfectionism is the first coexisting condition due to its natural intertwinement with the disorder itself. Thus, it will be deeply analyzed based on a paper published by the Australian Psychological Society in 2014 regarding perfectionism and anxiety as part of a combined series of coexisting conditions with and beyond anxiety.

Perfectionism has long been linked to an increased risk for anxiety, a connection that cannot simply be boiled down to a gut feeling. Perfectionism is about striving; it fosters feelings of chronic stress and unhappiness, and often leads to intense anxiety. The constant expectation to perform can also rapidly become mentally exhausting. There is a good chance that many adults could identify as having those perfectionistic tendencies. Paradoxically, anxiety and stress are well-known blockers in actual performance. This inability to allow for error is inherently flawed and contradictory.

2. Understanding Perfectionism

Due to the standards that are set, failing to meet these high targets can fill a perfectionist with feelings of incompetence, which can bring about severe anxiety and subsequently depression. Being filled with anxiety can also add to emotional dysregulation, life issues from relationships to work. Ensuring everything is in order can take up most of your time, leaving you with very little time for fun, enjoyment, and relaxation. Achievements often go unnoticed due to feelings of guilt that time was wasted and things were not achieved, and the circle starts afresh.

Each type of perfectionist may have these traits ingrained in them, something that tarnishes every single aspect of their life, or may have certain traits at home but not in sport, or vice versa. When rounded off, if you have issues with parts of your life and symptoms of anxiety, you may find that the cause of it is in the black and white haze of perfectionism that clouds your day-to-day activities.

Perfectionism is the constant striving for flawlessness, setting high standards, and being overly critical of oneself and one's place in the world. It is the belief that anything less than perfect will be, at worst, catastrophic and, at best, acceptable but not good enough. With these high standards for oneself, one can only expect these people to apply the same standards to others, causing friction and stress in relationships with family, friends, and colleagues. It is a common myth that perfectionism is the same as being successful or having high standards – this is not true.

Instead, perfectionists have impossible standards and a definition of what success truly is. Many people consider themselves to be perfectionists but may not understand what kind of perfectionism they have. There are many different types of perfectionism, with the three main types defined by psychologist Dr. Paul Hewitt.

2.1. Definition and Types of Perfectionism

Perfectionism can be defined as a multifaceted personality trait characterized by a striving for flawlessness and demanding standards for performance, accompanied by critical self-evaluations and concerns regarding others' evaluation or judgment. There are two primary dimensions of perfectionism: 1) perfectionistic strivings or adaptive perfectionism; and 2) perfectionistic concerns or maladaptive perfectionism. Striving for perfection in an adaptive way can lead to positive outcomes, including well-being. Unfortunately, rigid and critical self-standards cause logical discrepancies that promote maladaptive achievement emotions, such as fear of failure and anxiety. Perfectionism has been shown to be correlated with a host of negative outcomes including, but not limited to, low self-esteem, depression, hopelessness, anger, anxiety, and stress. Regulatory perfectionism in particular has been implicated in the etiology and maintenance of panic and anxiety.

Experts believe that perfectionism can contribute to mental illness and unhealthy behaviors. According to the theory of positive disintegration, improvement in one or more of these dimensions can lead to personal growth and transformation. This suggests that the development of perfectionism - and its subsequent prevention and resolution - could play a role in individual and societal betterment as well. The easiest way to treat mental illness is to prevent it from taking root in the first place.

2.2. Causes and Triggers of Perfectionism

A highly anxious temperament may provide the perfect breeding ground for the development of perfectionism. Similarly, Type A personalities, which are typically characterized by rigid adherence to deadlines, time constraints, and appointment schedules, may also be at risk of developing perfectionism due to their frequently imposed demands for efficiency and productivity. Additionally, several personality traits have also been linked to perfectionism. One such trait is conscientiousness, a trait typified by high levels of orderliness, self-discipline, and competence. Conscientious individuals engage in frequent goal-setting and often monitor their levels of performance to ensure their satisfaction with an end product. Such a regimented approach to performance and goal-oriented behavior, however, can catalyze perfectionism. In particular, a highly conscientious individual is at risk of developing pathological perfectionism when he or she begins to engage in exaggerated, over-ambitious, excessively self-critical, and inflexible striving concerning his or her performance. The interface between conscientiousness and self-criticality becomes important as perfectionism surfaces as the threshold of self-criticism crosses a certain point.

2.2. Causes and Triggers of Perfectionism. What circumstances or personality traits may cause the development of perfectionism? Although an exact or certain answer to this question remains challenging, evidence generally suggests that perfectionism may result from a combination of temperament, family, social, and interpersonal factors. In understanding these underlying perfectionistic factors, it becomes easier to appreciate how perfectionism and anxiety relate to each other. The same triggers and causes that lead to the development of perfectionism have also been associated with the onset and perpetuation of anxiety, suggesting that the two phenomena are intricately connected.

3. Understanding Anxiety

Symptoms of anxiety can manifest themselves in a real variety of ways, leading to a diverse range of both mental and physical symptoms. Mentally, sufferers may feel like they are losing control or impending doom is looming, and feel constant apprehension and restlessness, irritability, or increased sensitivity. This can then have a knock-on effect and cause physical symptoms like shaking or trembling, sweating, breathlessness, racing heartbeat, exhaustion and decreased immunity, and muscle tension. It's common for physical symptoms to be mistaken for medical problems in anxiety sufferers and vice versa because when anxiety is a constant presence in someone's life, it is always essentially bubbling under the surface, just waiting to be triggered into something more with the addition of (if only minor) stressors. Of course, all of this physical and mental discomfort then has an overall effect on the social life, choices, and activities of the person who experiences these thoughts and symptoms. The person may not take up work, pursue hobbies, or make close connections with others since they have difficulty completing goals or attempting new ventures. Conversely, the individual may immerse himself or herself in numerous activities, behaviors, or relationships to avoid feeling anxious.

Anxiety: What is it and what different disorders are there? Nobody can feel perfectly happy and relaxed all of the time, but if you are someone who regularly feels anxious and worries excessively and at length, then this could indicate that you have anxiety or an anxiety disorder. Anxiety disorders come in many forms and can have many effects on your everyday life if they are severe enough. The most common anxiety disorders include social anxiety, panic disorder, phobias, generalized anxiety disorder, separation anxiety, agoraphobia, specific phobias, and anxiety disorder due to a medical condition.

3.1. Types of Anxiety Disorders

An intolerance of uncertainty.

Performed motor actions that are not smooth or not functioning as they did prior to anxiety disorder.

Recurring, Intrusive, Highly Disturbing Thoughts coupled with a sense that what's happening isn't really happening.

ARE THERE DIFFERENTIATIONS BETWEEN TWO ANXIETY DISORDERS? There is some overlap between anxiety disorders, yes, but separation is ultimately maintained.

OCD (Obsessive Compulsive Disorder): This disorder is characterized by unusually amplified responses to those uncomfortable physical symptoms of keeping dirty hands, for example. The anxiety that is characteristically associated with dirt or disease becomes itself the problem.

Panic Disorders: Characterized by sudden feelings of intense terror. This can be paired with a feeling of detachment, or with a dread of dying without having lived one's life to the fullest.

Social Anxiety: Characterized by an irrational fear of embarrassment by those around you. An anxiety disorder not to be mistaken as simple shyness. Based on irrational fears of genuine catastrophe or serious ridicule caused by one's actions in social settings.

Generalized Anxiety: Characterized by the over-preoccupation with daily life causing one to worry to an almost pathological extent. Those who suffer from generalized anxiety are often unable to deal with poor performance on even those tasks which are objectively challenging.

When it comes to diagnosing an anxiety disorder, precision is paramount. Countless medical professionals, case workers, and laypersons compromise accuracy out of expediency. The pathology of perfectionism, paired with anxiety, amplifies the necessity to separate these many forms of universality. If one is to treat this disorder, understanding its specific form is indispensable. Below are the classifications of the dynamic distortions that constitute an anxiety disorder:

3.2. Symptoms and Effects of Anxiety

Anxiety's symptoms result in a surge of metabolic consequences. Anxiety takes a hefty toll on the body and mind with its common terrible mind-body shackles and its destructive impact on the immune system. The possible consequences are exhaustion, despondency and competitive issues. Rather than automatically warning us in danger, the common mental habits of anxious people reduce the likelihood of life's reality whenever they are perceived, imagined, or anticipated.

Anxiety is composed of three pieces: theme, emotions, and discernment. The unifying emotion of anxiety is rejection, and "stressed" people often experience it and may be unaware of it. Some people remain aloof in the face of a major life-crisis, while others are agitated by a single critical comment. Whether stress is internal as a concerned or external as a worrywart, the environment has a significant impact on the degree of shrinkage.

Anxiety is an intense fear or dread of anticipated events or experience of powerlessness that can occur on a level between problem-solving concern and paranoia. It is actually combined with tracking and avoiding presumed or real events, irritants or events. Despite a number of agreed symptoms including rumination, anticipatory affray, and the need to avoid or procrastinate getting started, anxiety is a multifaceted problem.

Anxiety is prevalent in our technologically advanced society. Sometimes, wedding cake meltdowns or final exams can cause more than just a little pressure. Anxiety occurs when a pending or future event is perceived to be life threatening. If these feelings are severe enough, the person impacted might not be able to carry out regular activities or be calm or comfortable. Anxiety is a normal expected response to the body experiencing threats. While this feeling is subjective, severe, continuous, or irrational fear can interfere with regular activities and perhaps lead to a range of physical symptoms.

4. The Perfectionism-Anxiety Connection

5. The Cycle of Perfectionism and Anxiety

Second, as will be discussed in a later blog post, anxiety can help bolster perfectionistic standards. Perfectionists carry around rigid standards about what must be at all times. Anxiety provides a threat to these individuals and so encourages them to adopt greater attention to detail and perfectionistic traits. Third, perfectionism leads to heightened anxiety and stress. When individuals are unable to meet their perfectionistic standards, a great deal of self-doubt arises within them. They are unable to accept that failure is a normal and inevitable part of life. The anxiety is managed by holding relentless standards and striving for perfection. By holding themselves to an impossible standard, they believe that they are avoiding and protecting themselves from painful and perceived catastrophic thoughts. This also leads to them to display avoidance behavior. The belief and the avoidance maintains the greater style of perfectionistic behavior.

In the last few blog posts, I discussed perfectionism and anxiety. There is a reciprocal relationship between perfectionism and anxiety. That is, they both cause and serve as an effect or symptom of the other. Thus, the two difficulties form a cycle. Many factors help to reinforce the cycle of perfectionism and anxiety. First, anxiety and perfectionism share a similar cognitive style. Perfectionism involves a rigid and rigidly held all-or-nothing standard of evaluation or perfection, whereas anxiety is characterized by rigid and rigidly held dichotomous evaluative beliefs. These beliefs divide experience into two distinct categories of good and bad.

6. Impact on Mental Health

One of the most challenging aspects of working with perfectionism is that it tends to have emotion dysregulating properties. This means that people with perfectionistic tendencies often feel a wide range of uncomfortable emotions including rejection, shame, and anxiety. This emotion dysregulation often makes perfectionism-driven individuals very difficult to work with, as therapy can easily feel like a game of whack-a-mole; whereby each negative emotion resolved just crops up again in a different form. Furthermore, many of these emotions have the same physiological activation of a lack of control situations which we see associated with anxiety. It is thereby not surprising that perfectionistic tendencies have been strongly linked with depression, anxiety-related disorders, and generalized anxiety in particular. In fact, anxiety appears to be potentially a symptom and a driver of certain subtypes of perfectionism. During the pandemic, studies indicate that it is associated with increased experiences of PTSD and social phobia.

According to Dr. Hewitt and many other researchers and mental health professionals, perfectionism is a major risk factor for anxiety and other forms of mental health distress. It's important to understand just how damaging perfectionism-induced anxiety can be to mental health. Anxiety will often worsen over time in the context of perfectionism. Many will begin to experience difficulties in settings outside of academia such as work and interpersonal relationships. In the absence of recovery, the risk of suicidal ideation or attempts also appears to be higher in those with perfectionism-related anxiety.

7. Breaking the Cycle: Strategies and Techniques

In addition to anxiety management tools, there are also strategies that can be utilized to break the cycle of perfectionism being described above. Try some of these strategies: set moderation goals for being perfect. This means giving oneself explicit permission to obtain marks of 85, 80, 70 or even 60 percent. Make a list of 20 things that one wants to accomplish and deliberately choose not to do several of them perfectly. Then go ahead and be less than perfect (see "toxic" rules for why this can be a good idea); try something new, where there's no hope of perfection yet: take up a new sport, join a singing group, try a new language; learn to laugh at mistakes, really punch holes in perfectionistic beliefs. For example, if one says or writes something that isn't perfect, she might say something like "Ha! There I go again, putting my foot in mouth!" Over time these kinds of light-hearted jibes help to undermine the toxic belief that one's worth depends on always being right and in control. Explore and challenge core beliefs about perfection: is the thought "I must be perfect" absolutely true?

You are not alone in experiencing the unwanted consequences of perfectionism. Many students report that perfectionism negatively affects their mental health and psychological well-being, increasing performance anxiety. In fact, perfectionism significantly predicts anxiety symptoms. This relationship is moderate and relatively consistent across different subscales of perfectionism (e.g., self-oriented, other-oriented, and socially prescribed). But the good news is that anxiety can be managed! Techniques and strategies (or self-help tools) to address and manage anxiety will be explored in a later section.

8. Cognitive-Behavioral Therapy (CBT) for Perfectionism and Anxiety

9. Mindfulness and Meditation Techniques

In some studies, people practicing mindfulness skills experience a reduction in their levels of clinical and nonclinical anxiety. When mindfulness is used as a therapeutic intervention, it can reduce the physical and psychological expressions of anxiety in an individual. Research shows a correlation between trait anxiety and the level of perfectionism an individual experiences. This means they can be used as a therapeutic intervention for reducing anxiety in someone with clinical perfectionism. Practitioners should look to advocate for the beneficial effects a holistic approach that practices both mental and physical techniques in tandem has. Practicing more physical self-care activities such as exercise could potentially decrease the effectiveness of any reduction in anxiety because of the underlying belief that productivity is connected to self-worth.

Mindfulness practices have demonstrated to be effective in promoting a reduction in psychological symptoms and an increase in physical benefits. These benefits make mindfulness practices a useful tool to improve mental well-being in perfectionism and anxiety. Mindfulness-based interventions preferentially address the present moment and practice non-judgment, acceptance, trust, and compassion. There is evidence that mindfulness may be associated with low levels of perfectionism. People who actively practice the self-compassion component in mindfulness-based practices become less concerned with failure and more resilient when faced with anxiety-inducing situations. Mindfulness-based practices (MBPs) have demonstrated a reduction in the intolerance of uncertainty and worry.

10. Setting Realistic Goals and Expectations

Perfectionists often struggle to set goals because they feel that the goals they set are either unattainable or they don't know the next step in the multi-step process that might lead to eventual attainment. If you find yourself plagued by such fears, try to accept (and even expect) some small failures along the way. It's far better to set small, achievable goals that make you feel productive and good about yourself every day than to set a large goal that inevitably feels further away with the passing of each day.

Setting realistic and attainable goals

Most senior leaders are results driven. They set performance goals, and they expect to see sustained and consistent results. But to set yourself up for healthy motivations, consider revisiting your goal-setting and the way you view your own success. When you evaluate whether you or the people working for you are successful, look at two things: 1. What were the people working for you asked to do? 2. Given what they were asked to do, what did they accomplish? Which measures should mean more to you? People often have an enormous amount of discretion over the things they choose to accomplish at work. Goals around innovation output are especially open to employees to over- or undercommit to. So if someone didn't accomplish what they set out to do, it may have been simply because they reached too high.

Outcome driven vs. Results driven thinking

11. Self-Compassion and Acceptance

Breaking Off the Circle of Perfectionism and Anxiety: A Self-Empathy Script A great amount of research has been dedicated to understanding the reason for its existence. However, this article focuses on a belief detailed by Tracy Martin's work in her book "The Confident Creative: Drawing to Free the Hand and Mind" (2008). Drawing from her experience and interviews with professional creatives from two sectors, music composition and commercial advertising, Martin found that perfectionism was a climate the professionals all lived and thrived in for several reasons, despite perfectionism being dismissed as a negative way of thinking whenever it was discussed.

5. Use the concept of pausing: When an action needs to be performed or a decision needs to be made, decide to take a few seconds to reflect on the choice to be made or modified, respecting several choices.

4. Use a gentler inner voice only with yourself: Look for ways to relate to your own perfectionism in an open-minded and curious way, externalizing its effects and seeing it as a separate part of your personality and your life.

3. Cultivate an understanding and clear perspective: Focus on the positive sides of your imperfections and the (unknown) back channels to success.

2. Remember you're only human: Consider cost-effective ways to problem-solve when things don't turn out as planned.

1. Offer yourself self-kindness: Cut yourself some slack by using a compassionate inner voice to talk about yourself; essentially, redirect negative thoughts away from you.

Self-compassion and mindfulness combined can support you in gently working with yourself through times of perfectionism and anxiety. Bringing mindfulness into perfectionism practices can help as well. An acceptance of one's perfectionism itself trickles into breaking the cycle of performing one's best, no more inner dialogue.

12. Building Resilience and Coping Skills

13. Challenging Perfectionistic Thoughts and Beliefs

One treatment that is particularly effective at helping people to learn more adaptive beliefs and reduce associated anxiety is cognitive restructuring (CR). In CR, you learn how to counteract cognitive distortions with more balanced, flexible thoughts. This new way of thinking can help clear space for more pleasant experiences; reducing perfectionistic thoughts can help you in relation to feeling less anxious. Helper Joe knows with this technique that he needs to help his reader start to see a different perspective on problems or on their general approach to goals as a very first step in beginning to feel differently. It is when they have the chance or capacity to also shift how they have learned over time to feel about trying to be 'perfect' at something.

Challenging perfectionistic thoughts and beliefs is a crucial part of breaking the cycle of perfectionism and anxiety. When you are anxious, you might experience a range of cognitive distortions or tricky thinking styles. Some of these are particularly common in perfectionism. For instance, you might often jump to conclusions, such as believing that something is a complete disaster or hopeless just because it's not perfect. Other perfectionistic thinking might include overgeneralizing or catastrophizing. For example, you might inadvertently transform specific problem behaviors or issues into some kind of character flaw or global loss. Perhaps you forget to complete something work-related and assume that no matter what you do or say, you might as well quit now. Or if you don't meet your own very high standards in a particular area of your life, it feels like the end of the world. Alternatively, it might be all or nothing thinking, and you think that if you just engage in negative thinking about yourself that you will be able to scare yourself into success.

14. Practicing Self-Care and Stress Management

Stress I Can Do Something About: How do you feel about this design? Fill in the blank and/or add any comments you would like to include. Examples: The source of stress in my life is mostly... What do I usually do about it? I try to...

How to Take Good Care of Ourselves: How do young people become happy and fulfilled caring people themselves? Start with nurturing their own well-being, practicing self-care, and managing our own stress. The gifts of self-care help us to grow stronger, are able to deal with the pressures in our practice, and can connect to that quiet still inside ourselves.

Self-care is important! Also, resource students in guidance and counseling services. The practitioner has permission to assist you with some stress management techniques that could come in handy to combat perfectionist anxiety and improve self-worth. In times of extreme stress, you can access the following supports: Emergency telephone counseling 24 hrs/day, 7 days/week - Crisis Response Centre - Mobile Crisis - Kids Help Phone if you are under 19. Other immediate phone numbers for students in distress: Ambulance 911 (if someone is physically hurt) or call Campus Safety - (for a first aid kit if you or another student is physically cut).

15. Social Support and Communication Skills

Numerous findings tell us that the social network of individuals, the quality of relationships, and the extent to which it can provide support in painful situations seem to be implicated in the degree of psychological well-being or the associated emotional states. The presence of people around us who can help us in times of need provides additional opportunities for how we (inter)act when we are overwhelmed by distress or are anxious, and this can certainly be an advantage against the harmful effects of anxiety and perfectionism. Communication at several levels builds a range of alternatives on how to cope with life's downs. It can assist in early detection, it can mobilize us to search for help, and ultimately it can facilitate access to another "wisdom" discreetly seated in the heads of our significant others, which may relate to showing new ways to look at the situation or new ways to deal with it.

Perfectionism and anxiety are not in any way incurable characteristics because support from the outside serves an important role in managing their effects. The clear and honest statement of Mrs. Jacobs in the quotation above may be good advice for many. There is a well-known correlation between explanatory style and well-being, in which optimists are on the healthier side. If we do not have the benefit of a natural tendency to an optimistic way of explaining the ups and downs of life, and if psychological counseling is not a passion, the best advice for managing the anxiety that stems from perfectionism is social support.

16. Physical Health and Well-Being

We exist in a society that values well-being, not just physical health. Well-being is broad enough to encompass a whole bunch of things and yet specific enough to offer defined outcomes for which we can work. The role of mental health is as important as physical health in determining our overall well-being. Mental illnesses (like anxiety, depression, bipolar disorders, PTSD, etc.) are agonizing and very distressing. They can eventually make us physically ill as well. The fourth aspect specifically mentioned in the NICE guidelines is "some physical health conditions". Just as anxiety and perfectionism are related, stress and physical health are also interrelated. Stress can cause physical health issues, and poor physical health can cause stress. Both result in a feedback loop.

If we are content with our current state of health, we cannot expect things to change or improve. Perfect health is a vague term that has as many ideal standards as there are people. This ambiguity can indicate that perhaps health and disease are not two entirely different compartments in the human body. Too narrow a focus on 'not being ill' can overlook the need to work equally hard at developing the ability to be in the best possible form, free of symptoms, pain, and emotional entanglements. The physical and the mental are interconnected in more ways than we can understand. Mental anxieties can lead to physical illness via the immune system's dysfunction. Similarly, physical illnesses like autoimmunity can underpin mental health issues like stress, anxiety, and depression.

17. The Role of Exercise and Nutrition

Although it is an important lifestyle habit to be aware of the inclusion of good nutrition in our day-to-day lives, too often, excessive attention to "trigger" foods and food groups can perpetuate the fear of consuming "bad" food with the belief that we are then "poisoning" our bodies. Instead of viewing a food as something that will help our performance as humans, some individuals can see it as something which can make or break our goals, whether they be aesthetic, fitness, or health related. Nutrients are the essential elements to fuel fat loss, increase muscle mass, improve physical performance, and keep our tissues and organs healthy. As the fuel required to generate energy to support our daily activities as well as help us recover from resistance training, nutrients play a key role in optimizing our functioning and recovery processes. Just as over-exercising can lead to burnouts, over-fixating about nutrient intake can trigger anxiety levels and possibly even harm future health. Aiming for an "intuitive eating" approach, where some basic rules are followed but there is no fear or anxiety towards food, is ideal.

In order to maintain physical health, it is absolutely critical that we exercise. Exercise has so many benefits to our physical body, including weight regulation, improved muscle health, maintaining the health of our cardiovascular system, and maintaining the health of our skin. Exercise also has profound benefits on our mental health, including improvement of mood, decreased anxiety levels, and improvement of cognitive function. With regard to our mood, exercise often directly activates the release of endorphins, hormones that are responsible for creating positive feelings and reducing the perception of pain. Endorphins act within the brain to reduce our awareness of pain as well as delivering a euphoric boost in mood, commonly known as a "runner's high." Regular physical exercise also decreases our levels of the stress hormone cortisol, resulting in a more relaxed feeling and decreased feelings of anxiety.

18. Sleep Hygiene and its Impact on Anxiety and Perfectionism

Disengagement is not always the healthful aspect of "I don't feel like doing anything" when it precedes or causes the problem. But often, finding one valued, valid reason as a productive foundation for getting out of bed regardless of the circumstances can, in itself, be empowering for some. Mindfulness of choices and habits can modify intention to live according to personal values of health even when there are feelings of having no worth. Women were reported as worried about sleep and partners, finance, drugs, and memories compared to men pre-medically unwell. Choosing "the tiniest bedtime distraction," morning awakening, and dozing during the day improves the level of optimal sleep with consistent well-being.

Sleep hygiene, anxiety, and perfectionism: why are they included? The repetition of this unit operation emphasizes the importance of sleep and the reciprocal relationship between sleep and psychological well-being. This demonstrates the importance of healthy sleep habits, which may be disrupted by afflictions such as circadian rhythm disorders and the disorders mentioned in Chapter 11. It does not matter which comes first: the psychological distress (and/or clinical diagnosis), sleep disorder, or the "bad" habits that interfere with good sleep and thus neuronutrition and emotional wellness. Interruption of the cycle is important, and care might include managing sleep-inhibiting thoughts, anxiety, and archaic, ill-informed but sometimes far too powerful hypnophobic beliefs.

19. Professional Help and Resources

If professional support that guides you through a specialized intervention isn't available to you, there are resources and self-help treatments available for download online. Always look for the resources that provide self-help treatment interventions that have some research evidence to support their effectiveness. "Many people who present to my clinic have already used a number of available online resources prior to coming in to see us," said clinical psychologist Dr. Stuart Norman, who specializes in treating anxiety disorders and other associated difficulties. A doctors' group in Canada called Opioid Prescribing Skills Assessment (OPSA) recently released evidence-based guidelines for treating insomnia in adults. These guidelines suggest that cognitive-behavioral therapy — an individualized program that people work through with a therapist's guidance — is the best first-line approach for treating insomnia that isn't caused by some other health problem. Cognitive-behavioral therapy is as effective as taking prescription sleep medications, and is more likely to help patients feel better over the long term as well.

Seeking professional help is the best option for treating severe cases of anxiety disorders and associated difficulties, including distress related to perfectionism. Look into seeing a mental health professional, who may specialize in treatment for anxiety, eating disorders, or mood disorders. Many people who struggle with anxiety disorders and related difficulties such as distress related to perfectionism don't receive treatment, whether because they don't expect help to be effective or don't think they need help. "Even if you may not recognize yourself as someone with an 'anxiety disorder,' if you're feeling down, overwhelmed, or you're perfectionistic and start avoiding things you used to enjoy, working with a professional skilled in treating anxiety or related difficulties can offer an opportunity to break these patterns," according to Dr. Elisa Nebolsine, a clinical psychologist specializing in treating anxiety-related conditions and disorders.

20. When to Seek Therapy or Counseling

You may also have used "brush-offs" or coping strategies that do not address the root cause for your pain or suffering. These "off the top" strategies may have included: shopping, alcohol and drugs in quantity or chronically, overeating, dieting, smoking, crazy dieting behaviors, and non-stop exercise. You may also have gotten as a way to ease your "pain". There is a way to a new life, but it is not by doing "off the top" things that reframe, pull, push or talk yourself, or others, into a sense of ease or well-being. All that path would get you would be to forget it, until it surfaces again and again to wake you from your sleep - in one shape or another. You may also have inherited aspects from your family that make continued struggle likely. In excising yourself from suffering, we will help you to remember something precious and to learn something new that might be strange unfamiliar at first, but in the end it would be based on truths known in your heart.

• When you find that you can't manage perfectionism or anxiety on your own, you are probably a prime candidate for professional help. Be smart - seek it out now. Don't wait for things to get so bad that you feel utterly out of control, or feel like you can't possibly keep living like you've been living. • Being human means struggling with stress, perfectionism, anxiety, limited coping strategies and slippage as you try to make changes. For these normal struggles, don't seek therapy. Everyone has some negative self-talk, tends to try to be a perfectionistic striver (sometimes or chronically), tends to be somewhat anxious rather than laid back, and gets into conflicts or disagreements with family members and others. These are all normal irritations in life. It's when you find that they are poisoning your life or the life of someone you love, when you feel like they're frittering your life away, and keeping you from living and relating authentically and powerfully that you need to seek professional help. Coming to the point where you seek professional help usually takes couples, men, moms or individuals about 10-20 years of "trying" on their own. You may have started seeking help from self-help books and then have gone on to personal growth group work such as DI or PDI (the now closed Diablo Institute or Pacific Diablo Institute), seminar series, body works, chiropractic, acupuncture, naturopathy, hypnotherapy, EMDR therapy, psychotherapy, etc.

21. Finding the Right Therapist or Mental Health Professional

You should also feel free to ask specific, practical questions about the therapy process. These might include, "How much does this cost?" "Are you in-network here?" "How long are the sessions?" and any other questions that you feel are relevant. People often meet with a few different professionals before they find someone they like. And if you go to a few sessions and don't like the person, feel free to look for a different therapist. There are many different styles of therapy. Cognitive-Behavioral Therapy (CBT) is often a good choice for people who struggle with perfectionism and anxiety. However, I have worked with some people for whom a different form of therapy has been a better fit. Some therapists will describe the approaches that are best supported by evidence (or "research-proven" therapies). Other therapists choose not to talk about this. In my experience, this choice doesn't always reflect their skills as a therapist.

When choosing a therapist or mental health professional, there are a few things to consider. First and foremost, it's important to find someone who you feel comfortable talking to. Considering the role perfectionism plays in anxiety disorders, the therapist should have experience in treating perfectionism. The therapist should also be well-versed in treating anxiety disorders. For some people, it is especially helpful to work with a professional who has experience in treating individuals who have struggled with similar issues. Unfortunately, not every therapist will be able to meet these criteria. During a free initial consultation, you might ask them directly if they have ever treated someone who is struggling with the same issue that you're struggling with.

22. Online and Teletherapy Options

At more basic levels, they are flexible and possible to attend even for people with busy working routines or caring for children. Some work very quickly to allow those with mental health struggles to have preliminary advice in as soon as 6 weeks. They can also involve other methods of healing as well as personal counselling, such as with those who participate in offerings from online relationships who have access to collective group and contact support. Digital forums provide access to countless self-help books, articles, videos, and mental health resources. Many will provide practical and efficient coping strategies or insights or information into the way the patient feels and what kind of treatment will be best for them either personally or generically. Many were also covered on measuring FS and improving self-esteem and even better being free of charge for the patient.

Counselling and therapy are often two immediate decisions faced by sufferers of anxiety. Unfortunately, because many perfectionists do not realize they have a psychological or mental issue, their first port of call will likely be pursuing help for their anxiety. Online and teletherapy options are becoming increasingly available, from NHS or faith-based offerings to competitive commercial sites.

23. Support Groups and Peer Networks

Being among others who feel as we do helps us draw courage from the collective wisdom and strength of the group. We can notice that the problems and the feelings they provoke are not our fault, and may find it easier to talk openly and honestly. What we talk about in groups is confidential, and a facilitator will manage the discussion to keep it safe. We stick to what is happening now, in the present. We do not give advice, 'fix' participants, or refer them to services. Group memory – together we can piece together events. Members are not compelled to tell it all, but the truth always comes out in a small group sooner or later! If someone is concerned about another participant, we ask them to speak to that person and say why.

Support groups and peer networks can offer valuable opportunities for talking about the challenges of perfectionism and anxiety and finding out what might – or might not – work for others in similar situations. This can make us feel understood and less isolated, and reduce the intensity of our suffering. But connection can also bring other less obvious benefits. When we share a story – a real, lived experience – our brain responds not only with understanding and compassion, but also with oxytocin, the "compassion hormone," which increases trust and reduces fear. So, when we connect and feel felt, not only does our anxiety decrease, but we also feel braver.

24. Conclusion: Embracing Imperfection and Growth

While we obviously can't change our thinking pattern overnight (no matter what the self-help books or gurus might claim), taking small, baby steps towards that growth mindset on a more regular basis can be incredibly helpful. When we catch ourselves entertaining thoughts that are fueled by perfectionism, we can try to become the objective observer rather than wire ourselves up to a lie detector test. We can try to talk to ourselves like a friend would talk to us if we were to confide in them. Finally, we can come to our own unique behavioral conclusions. What does healthy risk-taking 'decision-making' look like? Sometimes performing spontaneously, occasionally second-guessing, switching up established routines and rituals or demonstrating curiosity and unbound potential with no room for excessive withdrawals.

Our culture doesn't always make it easy for perfectionists not to struggle with anxiety. To some extent, we should all probably strive for performance that is good enough rather than perfect. But we should also be compassionate to ourselves when our performance isn't perfect. Growth is a win-lose game. While we may get better at certain things faster than others, there will always be someone who is better than us at the things that are important to us. The only way to not end up disliking ourselves and being unhappy is to be kind to ourselves when we don't meet our personal standards. Just because part of us is suffering doesn't mean that part of us is right. We are more than just our thoughts and feelings. Embracing a growth mindset can help us gradually shift our perspective.

The Relationship Between Anxiety and Perfectionism: Understanding and Breaking the Feedback Loop

1. Introduction to Anxiety and Perfectionism

The bidirectional influences of emotional disorders and attitudes towards oneself and the world have been relatively well studied for depression. Given that anxiety and perfectionism stresses serve similar motivational and emotional functions, it would be expected that anxiety impacts perfectionism, and vice versa. However, in a major critique of the literature, McMahon and Kotowarich suggest that much of the research on the anxiety-perfectionism relationship has been atheoretical. As such, they provide an etiological framework for anxiety, one which encompasses vulnerability factors such as perfectionism alongside precipitating stressors such as increasing academic pressure. They describe perfectionistic self-feeds which simultaneously maintain the cycle of anxiety and perfectionism relationships, making them likely to transdiagnostically maintain any and all anxiety disorders.

Anxieties and intense self-doubts are common experiences for most people striving for success in a given domain. Whether footballers before a game, students writing exams, or professionals sharing presentations with clients, fears of making mistakes, not doing well enough, or disappointing others can be highly distressing. For a not insignificant portion of the population, the need to be perfect can become central to their identity. In the literature, perfectionism is conceptualized as the relentless striving for flawlessness and perfection, accompanied by critical evaluations of all personal achievements and deep concerns regarding public recognition. Moreover, high degrees of perfectionism are related to the perpetuation of anxiety disorders, such as obsessive-compulsive disorder and social anxiety. Considering that anxiety itself is one of the most frequent psychological disorders and global mental health, it becomes crucial to understand and intervene in the perfectionism-anxiety relationship.

2. The Interplay Between Anxiety and Perfectionism

Refined research from cross-sectional and longitudinal perspectives lends support for a reciprocal influence of perfectionism and anxiety, along with strong neurocognitive, biological, and epigenetic pathways in the etiology and maintenance of these maladaptive pathways. It appears to increase the attention given to mistakes in a task, as well as magnify the self-perception of the seriousness of mistakes. It is, therefore, not the mere presence of perfectionism or anxiety, much less their individual effects in relation to low-functioning or high-performance decrements, but instead the interaction of the two dynamically fueling their amplification that appears to lead to increased pathology and risk for both anxiety and perfectionism.

Decades of research have investigated whether anxiety precedes and drives the development of perfectionistic tendencies, or whether perfectionistic tendencies give rise to and amplify anxiety. This dynamic relationship between anxiety and perfectionism conjures to mind a pair of production and reception lines working simultaneously, each responding and presenting its offshoot of the other—both influencing and, in turn, being influenced by the output of the other. Broadly, perfectionism seems to occur in response to and amplify anxiety. It is important to draw a parallel here with obsessive-compulsive conditions, especially given that there is a clinical consensus in differentiating between a positive, adaptive form of perfectionism and an unhealthy, obsessive pursuit of flawlessness that involves constant self-criticism and the setting of unrealistic standards. Anxiety is related to the compulsion of stopping, checking, and correcting, in a similar sense that is characteristic of people with obsessionality, while perfectionism now takes the forefront as a focus of attention and driven efforts. Both constellations are then closely aligned with more general human qualities of responsibility and guilt.

2.1. Anxiety as a Driver of Perfectionism

Anxiety can be a key driver that leads and reinforces the perfectionism affliction in a feedback loop. An accurate working definition of perfectionism also includes anxiety as a core principle because one must be preoccupied with issues about achieving flawless standards within their own work. Perfectionism is to be present with a checklist of things, fleshing out anxiety at every stop or unattained destination. The desire to achieve only the best ideals leads also to the maximal amount of error and anxiety concerning personal control over the situation. Very rigid standards for performance and work directly connect to a belief in one's inefficacy to handle any possible failure, exponentially equating the achievement of these high goals to 'life or death' stakes. Either performance standards will be met in perfection (e.g. maintaining control over situations) and personal fears/existential uncertainties will be reduced temporarily, or the standards will not be met and uncontrolled situations and disaster will surely visit.

While it is not difficult to observe outwardly the products of perfectionism (e.g. recurrent and intrusive terminal doubt; 'crystallised role' perfectionism), the causes of perfectionism remain elusive. In this relationship between perfectionism and anxiety, it is somewhat intuitive for some to infer that perfectionists are the product of unreasonable levels of anxiety. They are, in other words, neurotic individuals who simply worry too much about the wrong things. It is, however, quite another matter to suggest that those predisposed to perfectionism may find their existing anxieties reinforced and internalised more readily than non-perfectionists. By absorbing their critical feedback in a perfectionistic register, not only does anxiety become more prominent and pronounced, but perfectionism may more closely resemble a dissociable and potentially chronic stressor that becomes inaccessible to reduction through mere reduction in the feedback loop: the relationships between flourishing and thriving consistent with perfectionism and other internalised disorder.

2.1 - Anxiety as a Driver of Perfectionism

2.2. Perfectionism as a Contributor to Anxiety

There are three general ways in which perfectionism can contribute to the experiences of anxiety. The first discloses the immense pressures that perfectionistic self-standards place on individuals. Moreover, that these pressures, once in place, are hard to ever fully resolve. The second reflects the accumulation of desired outcomes in the future. If the pressure described earlier is the pressure to get things right (but no real pressure to avoid the emotional consequences of getting things right). The final contribution to future anxiety is from a developing habit of questioning and undermining past successes. In particular, anxiety about not meeting such an insidious standard is difficult to challenge because refutation is anchored in past thinkings and past states of mind, both of which are invariable.

The findings of the prior section may help to explain why more intense states of anxiety precipitate and exacerbate perfectionism. It should be noted that anxiety is fueled by perfectionism, and it is not likely to be an innate problem for perfectionists. Namely, other experiences, such as falling short of one's standards or ruminating about attaining them, are likely responsible for these higher state anxiety responses in external validation negative feedback conditions. The heightened state anxiety scores, in the present study, are consistent with those found in previous research, which demonstrates the tight feedback loop between perfectionism and anxiety. In turn, since pre-existing anxiety is uninformative about scores on the perfectionism scale or those for the external standards mandate measure, it seems likely that perfectionism contributes to anxiety levels.

3. Psychological Theories and Research on Anxiety and Perfectionism

Shumaker and Duvdevany (2008) suggest that perfectionism may be one way that children develop generalized anxiety, based on relevant empirical findings. Thus, perfectionistic thinking style is associated with excessive fears such as separation anxiety, social anxiety, shyness, depression, and feelings of loneliness, mainly because the child experiences such high levels of self-doubt that they perceive their social environment to be threatening, as they are convinced that they are not "good" enough to justify how much they are expecting from others in the way of support and reassurance, with dire consequences if the others don't comply. In turn, attachment difficulties have been found to predict high perfectionism in children. A few research studies have identified a correlation between abnormally high anxiety levels and abnormally high perfectionism levels. Most researchers' findings suggest that this relationship is far from perfect, but that the two conditions are nevertheless linked. Alternatively, a 'split keys' effect sometimes occurs where individuals display one condition more so than the other, particularly in women.

Psychological researchers and theorists see interesting connections between anxiety and perfectionism, proposing that one leads to and sustains the other. This section will present evidence from psychological theory and empirical research into the nature and connection between these two concepts, how they interact and exacerbate each other to form a negative feedback loop which contributes to considerable distress. Perfectionism can be understood using a cognitive-behavioral perspective which suggests that the appraisal of the importance of one's actions, behavior, and performance is altered in a number of ways. Research into the causes of high self-expectations, particularly to do with perfectionism, also provides a link between anxiety and perfectionism. Attachment theory provides another means by which the relationship between anxiety and perfectionism can be understood.

3.1. Cognitive-Behavioral Perspective

1) Both perfectionism and anxiety are characterized by the presence of maladaptive cognitive factors such as cognitive distortions in thinking and belief systems that tend to perpetuate the level of both perfectionism and anxiety. 2) Perfectionism results in a range of maladaptive behavioral strategies that serve to maintain high levels of perfectionism (e.g., 'avoidance' of failed tasks; 'over-analysis' of performance), and because of cognitive feedback, this maintenance occurs not solely as a result of reduced chance to disconfirm beliefs about failing, but also relative to the secondary feedback that is often associated with these behaviors (e.g., feelings of reduced/avoided interpersonal evaluation). 3) Therefore, the unhelpful behavioral strategies that perfectionists engage in, as a result of their endorsement of the rigid clinical belief systems, serve to help maintain their high levels of anxiety in various situations, raising the risk that for those more anxious individuals these strategies could potentially facilitate the experience of poor mental health and depression. In testing the model in social anxiety disorder, students have found that perfectionism was significantly associated with the total number of safety behaviors, and these behaviors statistically mediated the relationship between self-critical threat and social anxiety symptoms accounting for a third of the variance. It is also has been hypothesized that interventions should focus on decreasing the importance of the perceived consequences of making a mistake, rather than just the frequency of

safety behaviors, as has been suggested in CBT for anxiety disorders.

Numerous reviews have been written providing details of cognitive-behavioral formulations of generalized anxiety disorder and social phobia. In the current section, we provide a brief framework for the relationship between perfectionism and anxiety, from the cognitive-behavioral perspective. We make reference to this work to illustrate four interdependent maintained by cognitive and behavioral processes. It is by our self and RQ that has suggested the potential widespread applicability of the principles of this model to other anxiety disorders. The formulation work also have tested between the psychological loci.

3.2. Attachment Theory

In clinical populations and in the extreme end of non-clinical populations, insecurities about the accessibility of emotional support are often linked with being more self-critical and less self-compassionate. This might be because emotional support from others generalizes onto the self, whereby those with more secure attachments believe they are valuable (i.e., self-compassionate) and thus do not need to harp on their imperfections. In contrast, those who are not convinced of their supporters' continued availability are more inclined to engage in so-called self-soothing strategies, including self-criticism (i.e., less self-compassionate) to regulate their internal states. In this way, viewpoints from attachment theory can extend the understanding of the relationship between anxious attachment orientations, anxieties about emotional threats, and related self-critical appraisals in perpetuating emotional distress.

A central tenet of attachment theory is that early relational experiences, and the attachment patterns they engender, become generalized across developmental domains. That is to say, a secure history with attachment figures generally leads to a sense of safety, secure self-concept, and effective regulation (and repair) of emotion in self and others. This impels the individual's exploration and autonomy. In contrast, insecure attachment patterns arise from difficulty finding care and support in caregivers when needed, and cause disruptions in the self-regulation of affect. For example, anxious attachment orientations may manifest as hypervigilance and hyper-regulation in an attempt to restore attachment-related emotions. This feeds into a continued reliance on altered regulatory strategies coupled with hypervigilance about emotional threats (i.e., perfectionism).

4. Impact on Mental Health and Well-Being

Now is a perfect time to research the relationship between anxiety and perfectionism. The more we understand about this relationship, the better we will be able to understand the varied presentations of and the best strategies for ameliorating mental health challenges. It is time we examined whether the feedback loop suggested by Llera and Newman might extend to the perfectionism-anxiety interface. This, in turn, could highlight features of anxiety and perfectionism to target in treatment and/or support clinics, in terms of maintaining distress and dysfunction. Given the problems with comorbidity and those connected directly with the perfectionism-anxiety interface, so many individuals face, such targeted programs would fill a useful gap. Consequently, in this study, measures of both anxiety and perfectionism were administered at the same time. For the client group and for the anxious controls currently receiving treatment for their anxiety difficulties, measures of both anxiety and perfectionism were administered at the same time.

Connections between generalized anxiety and perfectionism have been observed in those with anxiety disorders and in counseling literature on coping with the stress of academic perfectionism. Both typically anxious individuals and those with OCD tend to have highly inflated standards for performance and perfectionistic cognitive and behavioral patterns, as well as a critical evaluation.

Individuals with an anxiety disorder exhibit both socially-prescribed and self-oriented perfectionism to a greater degree than healthy controls, suggesting that perfectionism may also play a role in anxiety maintenance. Clinical observations and some self-report studies also suggest that self-oriented perfectionism and perfectionistic strivings are related to self-doubts, anxiety or depression, and distressing intrusive thoughts or rumination in non-clinical populations. Furthermore, anxiety relating to the pursuit of a perfectionistic standard increases after the onset of such intrusive thoughts.

4.1. Anxiety Disorders

In addition to contributing to common negative emotions experienced by clients with anxiety, perfectionism has been found to predict the development of the disorder. In a large sample of 632 adult New Zealanders, perfectionism was identified as the strongest univariate predictor of the development of OCD, generalized anxiety disorder (GAD), social phobia, stage fright, cardiac phobia, and marriage phobia over a 12-month period. In a large sample of Dutch and Flemish adolescents, the adaptive dimension of perfectionism, personal standards, was found to predict an increase in obsessive-compulsive symptoms beyond the effects of environmental and common genetic influences. Additionally, both personal standards and maladaptive perfectionism were found to predict increases in depressive symptoms.

Anxiety and perfectionism not only occur together, but also appear in the same individual, causing a considerable amount of distress and impairment. They have also been identified as central maintaining factors across a number of anxiety disorders. Although interventions are typically discussed in terms of separate maintaining factors, it is evident that perfectionism is likely to contribute to the maintenance of anxiety-related difficulties. Therefore, interventions for anxiety disorders have been adapted to include attention to the reduction of perfectionism. This is achieved by addressing the negative self-evaluations and fear of negative evaluation held by perfectionists, while also attending to their perfectionistic standards and low self-compassion. These factors may negatively impact levels of self-efficacy, which is another cognitive maintaining factor. The faulty appraisal of fears by perfectionists may lead to difficulties in reducing and tolerating physiological sensations, as the perfectionist may interpret these fears as highly threatening and believe that they "can't cope." This perpetuates the cycle of anxiety. We discuss the complex interactions of these maintaining factors that may hinder recovery from anxiety across various presentations. We do this by detailing a graduated, sequential case study that links together perfectionism, social anxiety, panic disorder, post-traumatic stress disorder (PTSD), obsessive-compulsive disorder (OCD), and health anxiety.

4.2. Obsessive-Compulsive Disorder (OCD)

There is much to say on this subject due to the way that perfectionism influences other core symptoms of OCD. To find out more, researchers delved into everything they could find on perfectionism and OCD with people experiencing the contamination fears and washing compulsions or those with the fear of harming others or sexual thoughts. They found that tried and tested methods of understanding perfectionism were not helpful when it came to developing a model that explained how perfectionism contributes to OCD. The way in which perfectionism affects symptoms seems to be the key in explaining why individuals with OCD who are perfectionistic face such specific difficulties.

OCD is perpetuated by four psychological processes: perfectionism and the pursuit of certainty, thought-action fusion (belief that negative thoughts may lead to negative events, not just facilitate them), inflated responsibility and over-importance of thoughts. Perfectionism and the pursuit of certainty play key roles in the development and maintenance of obsessive-compulsive disorder (OCD) symptoms. The importance of perfectionism in OCD has led researchers to devise measures of "clinical perfectionism", with items relating to the pursuit of certainty. Counter-intuitively, perfectionism is also more strongly related to and observed in those experiencing obsessions characterized by themes of responsibility for future events (e.g. harm being caused to others) and certainty-related compulsions, than it is to those experiencing symmetry and order obsessions with ordering and counting compulsions.

4.3. Depression

Further investigation is required to explore the impact of such interventions and justify the links outlined; however, it is hypothesized that broadening the approach will help improve understanding of the considerable complexity involved. Modifying each common component will help individuals undergoing intervention to address the vulnerability factors, adopting a more proactive coping response and break the emotional exhaustion-feedback loop.

In discussing maintenance of depression, it is evident through multiple pathways that the negative impact of self-evaluative perfectionism and anxiety when left misunderstood and untreated has the strong potential to become cumulative. Small incremental self-evaluative changes may convert initial negative vulnerability to a depression diagnosis, eventually culminating in an even worse prognosis. The separate pathways in relation to the consideration of generalized perfectionism and specifically purging behavior, as well as the clinical decisions outlined for motivational interviewing, assisted in tailoring a multimodal treatment plan. Here, the same or similar components of the form outlined in Bandura's multicomponent model are actively targeted as they share relevance to both active client symptoms and the model discussed.

An examination of the pathways leading to the onset of depressive symptoms is consistent with the dual activation of perfectionism and anxiety vulnerability described in the response to the implications model of depression. Disorders informed but not formalized into a depression diagnosis are also vulnerable to experiencing the same issues associated with perfectionism and anxiety given that massive amounts of symptoms are shared with those formally ending with depression diagnoses.

The integrated model of the anxiety-perfectionism relationship can similarly be applied to the discussion of the vulnerability, onset, and maintenance factors in relation to depression. The two geometric assessment pathways outlined render an individual's physical and emotional health uniquely at risk of the onset of depression, independent of any formal anxiety disorder diagnoses. Referring to the integrated models first, it is clear that both general perfectionism and anxiety are equally positioned at the center, for their interaction extensively contributes to vulnerability. This process may explain why significant comorbidity has been documented between depression and anxiety, as well as disorders characterized by perfectionism also present with anxiety symptoms.

5. Recognizing the Signs and Symptoms of Anxiety and Perfectionism

Depending on our individual psychological tendencies, personality, and general emotional baseline, these two distressing experiences may compound over time when they coexist. Left unchecked, both on their own and especially in tandem, anxiety and perfectionistic thinking have the power to decimate any potential for happiness or contentedness we might feel, if such potential wasn't already thwarting daily. Changes in acting out or in internal or mental state can act as warning signs that a person is struggling for any number of reasons or issues. Helping people who are experiencing signs of distress is an area where we can be seen as effective and supportive collaborators. Because longer distress has an enduring impact on the nervous system, it is most helpful for everyone involved to get them through it as soon as possible.

Living in an anxiety-based culture can make it difficult to recognize when anxiety has become pervasive—indistinguishable from personality traits and individual habits—or when anxious responses are in excess of their triggering stimuli, making even mundane activities feel difficult, out of reach, or pointless. However, the pervasive, all-encompassing nature of anxiety makes it difficult to ignore in its most severe presentations. Symptoms of perfectionism, on the other hand, may result from a series of seemingly disconnected and even positive or productive thought processes. This allows perfectionism to "go under the radar" for many years, escalating unnoticed over time as the ever-looming threat of not meeting one's own expectations and fears of failure compound over time.

6. Breaking the Feedback Loop: Strategies and Interventions

Improve attitudes toward mistakes. One approach to reducing the negative emotional experiences of failure might be to target the relatively irrational beliefs that are characteristic of perfectionism. Cognitive-behavioral techniques for modifying beliefs about perfectionism and perfectionistic cognitions, in general, can disrupt the unhelpful resistance to acknowledging and confronting areas of concern, that is a feature of experiential avoidance. Bergman suggests such strategies in the treatment of eating-disordered clients. Hayes proposes exposure techniques that involve "explicitly admitting what bothers [clients] the most... only when bothering has been fully experienced in context,... a search for imperfections begins" that is followed by the instruction to "own up to it."

Given the mutually influential nature of anxiety and perfectionism, traditional anxiety-reducing interventions may also indirectly aid in ameliorating both issues. For example, cognitive restructuring techniques may reduce positive worry related to goal-attainment and achievement in perfectionistic individuals. One study similarly found evidence that clinical cognitive-behavioral therapy administered for the treatment of obsessive-compulsive disorder concurrently reduced both anxiety and perfectionistic symptoms. However, directly fostering a desire for change, self-efficacy, and belief in the possibility for improvement can be highly beneficial for breaking the feedback loop, particularly in populations for those clinicians are not equipped to comprehensively manage both clinical anxiety and disordered perfectionism. Therefore, while the reduction of anxiety will likely assist in reducing the "perfection" motivation, it is also critical for individuals to regain the "action" dimension of goal setting that perfectionism has impeded. Toward this end, the following suggestions may be of assistance: improve attitudes toward mistakes; adopt mindfulness-based practices to reduce experiential avoidance; set process goals; adopt alternative goal constructs; and consider constructive action-based coping strategies.

Strategies and Interventions

6.1. Cognitive Restructuring Techniques

Reappraisal falls within the tradition of cognitive-behavioral therapy, and functional magnetic resonance imaging research suggests it has been successful in reducing worry and increasing executive functions in generalized anxiety disorder. Reappraisal is a cognitive restructuring intervention that all fit within a classification system that examines when/why situations are appraised in ways that are detrimental to our physical or mental well-being. The techniques have been divided into two broad categories of intervention that teach an individual to either reduce the effect of maladaptive appraisals on well-being or they teach an individual to control and modify those same maladaptive appraisals. The author contends that practitioners might do well to incorporate both types of reappraisal interventions since together they would give an individual greater resilience against maladaptive cognitive processes.

Given the evidence of cognitive bias and its difficulty to treat, researchers sought out the underlying mechanisms that would be more effective in changing the cognitive processing style. Cognitive restructuring techniques all have the same aim: to challenge and modify the anxiety or perfectionism-driven cognitive appraisals that are presumed to maintain the respective maladaptive cognitions. Research has shown that cognitively-based techniques effectively change rumination, cognitive flexibility, evaluative feedback, and cognitive appraisal. In doing so, cognitively-based techniques decrease the level of cognitive bias that maintains ill-being as well as the intensity of the resulting ill-being. Researchers would argue that the ultimate aim of using cognitive techniques is to reduce the strength with which someone perceives anxiety and worry as a credible source of information.

6.2. Mindfulness and Acceptance-Based Approaches

Mindfulness is closely related to acceptance, through the process of appraising our current psychological experience without avoiding, suppressing, trying to change, or escape it. Mindfulness and acceptance overlap significantly; some authors consider them so overlapping that they often discuss them within the context of a 'participatory, experiential approach to pain, distressing emotions and suffering'. It has been argued that mindfulness-specific therapeutic protocols pay more attention to the training of mindful awareness and the development of acceptance, while the general mindfulness-based therapies mainly focus on psychoeducation, training in acceptance, and education in mindfulness. Mindfulness interventions aim to enhance awareness and self-regulation practices to promote self-knowing and self-care behaviors, while self-compassion-based interventions attempt to stimulate a more supportive and friendly posture towards oneself, coping with perceived personal inadequacies in a compassionate rather than perfectionistic way. Acceptance-based interventions have been found to help individuals with perfectionistic tendencies to reduce their avoidance and promote effective inadequate self-schemas. Thus, exercises that explicitly target the acceptance of perceived personal inadequacies may help to interrupt the process of excessive goal pursuit and evaluation. More explicit evidence for the use of acceptance-based interventions in the context of perfectionism is lacking, although evidence for their use in anxiety-based disorders is positive.

Complementing the IP views, the remainder of the section will introduce mindfulness and acceptance-based strategies. Compared with the performance-approach IP model, mindfulness approaches break the link between anxiety and perfectionism where it starts: the valuation of the goal. Mindfulness, broadly speaking, is about being present. It is not about trying to clear the mind of thought, nor is it about making the mind blank. Instead, it is about noticing when the mind wanders, which it will, and gently, without judgment, bringing the focus back to the present moment. In terms more relevant to the present context, perfectionism and anxiety are about the future, such as constantly worrying about what might go wrong, or furiously trying to solve the associated difficulties. Mindfulness-based approaches suggest that practicing being present might also help us become more accepting of the inherently uncertain nature of the future, including allowing such worries and 'what-ifs' to come and go in their own time, not getting tangled in them in the process. The popularity of mindfulness is reflected in its extension to conceptualizations such as self-compassion and more general acceptance/well-being therapies.

6.3. Setting Realistic Goals and Expectations

To establish what realistically attainable goals are, it is important to reframe perfectionistic standards and aspirations. Paul Hewitt and colleagues argue that perfectionism is less about the pursuit of high standards per se and more about holding maladaptive evaluations of the self in response to not completing high standards. Simply setting for oneself more realistic achievements or aspirations is not likely to be entirely satisfying, as perfectionistic individuals may evaluate themselves as being imminently capable of achieving the higher standard. Instead, strive for standards and aspirations that are aligned with one's level of capability and skill. A commitment to being more compassionate to and maintaining realistic expectations of yourself should serve as the foundation of this change. In doing so, individuals may find that the pursuit of their goals is less anxiety relieving.

At the heart of perfectionism-driven anxiety is a lack of clarity surrounding what exactly sets an "attainable goal". This ambiguity makes it difficult to set realistic expectations and self-monitor adherence to these expectations. Dismissing the importance of effectively articulated goals, proponents of the Pygmalion effect argue that the manner and timing in which goals are enacted have a significant and morphogenic influence on the probability of goal achievement. This suggests that if there is a lack of clarity around the formulation of the goal, one is likely to set a vague and overly challenging goal. For those looking to minimize unwanted stress via setting attainable goals, guidance on determining what "attainable" means and looks like is needed. Here, distressing levels of perfectionism may be better managed indirectly, via adaptive goal-setting.

7. Counseling and Therapy Approaches

Outside of mainstream psychological therapies such as cognitive and behavioural therapies, there are some theoretical orientations and therapies that support this content by their strong emphasis on self-acceptance and self-compassion. Jungian therapy, humanistic therapies such as the person-centred approach or gestalt therapy, 12-step approaches, and existential approaches such as logotherapy. In addition to this, mindfulness-based approaches are very effective. Research shows that these therapies can all help with the effects of anxiety and perfectionism if the deeper elements of less compassionate self evaluations and belief systems are impacting upon the individual's ability to be in the world in a more satisfying manner.

Much has been made in the literature of how it's easy, if not entirely probable, that individuals experiencing anxiety and perfectionism lack the very skills necessary to feel better. Initial efforts around behaviour change can simply get caught in perfectionistic, negative feedback loops. Modifying unhelpful coping strategies directly or bluntly telling individuals they "should" change their behavior tends to be rejected or simply ignored, ultimately driving extreme self-criticism which burrows into anxiety. However, some psychological therapies, in particular cognitive-behavioral, are proving effective and this is why it is often worth giving things a try anyway, in many cases, remaining open minded and willing to experiment and see what happens can be quite helpful.

Counselling and therapy approaches

7.1. Cognitive-Behavioral Therapy (CBT)

CBT also can lead to a reduction in perfectionism through behavioral interventions. As previously outlined, several theories posit that a central driver for maintaining perfectionist beliefs is the presence of safety behaviors. With the right treatment approach, perfectionists may be coaxed to give up their safety behaviors and learn that the perceived 'worst' will not eventuate. Additional behavioral interventions used in CBT could potentially be used to foster other skills critical to undermining the anxious pattern maintained by the reciprocal relationship between perfectionism and anxiety. For example, behavioral interventions can be used to improve the client's distress tolerance and self-soothing abilities—skills that may be particularly important for reducing subjective anxiety.

Cognitive-behavioral therapy (CBT) may be particularly effective at addressing the relationship between anxiety and perfectionism because it intentionally targets both cognitions and behaviors. Cognitive restructuring techniques can be employed to challenge an individual's thoughts related to perfectionistic beliefs and expectations. For example, the assumption that 'flaws are not acceptable' may be countered with evidence that all individuals have various imperfections that are simply part of being human. The application of exposure-based techniques within a cognitive-behavioral framework can also be used to address core fears related to performance failure and profound rejection. This might look like an individual slowly exposing themselves to mistakes and imperfections that they have previously sought to avoid. As such, CBT interventions can target the impact of perfectionism on anxiety by helping clients to develop a variety of additional coping skills and adaptive strategies for managing core fears (e.g., if I make a mistake, I'll be seriously rejected).

7.2. Dialectical Behavior Therapy (DBT)

Overall, DBT proceeds in a stage-based approach and uses a multi-modal, or Zen-style, philosophy. The focus in the early stages of therapy is increasingly analytical and focuses on supporting behavior change through decreasing negative coping strategies and distress tolerance. DBT therapists focus on specific therapy goals to follow through with several therapeutic interventions, including the use of crisis survival strategies, teaching people to develop distress tolerance skills in session, ideas for building structure in a person's life, and ways to acquire and maintain a sense of mindfulness. As members more consistently regulate suicidal behavior and self-introduce more positive coping skills, individual treatment intensity is titrated down. Once the person is less overwhelmed and has fewer crises, the unbearable urges and impulses decrease. DBT reaches its ultimate goal of helping the person create a life worth living - one where the person can try things, explore, build new skills, and apply effective coping strategies.

Francism, a popular approach for working with individuals struggling with both anxiety and perfectionism, consists of traditional cognitive-behavioral strategies (e.g. exposure, cognitive restructuring, and behavioral experiments). While DBT has been criticized for commodity-driven dilutions, the evidence base has grown and an increasing number of randomized control trials have demonstrated DBT's efficacy for a range of problems. Further, many have emphasized how DBT incorporates a focus on interpersonal effectiveness and emotion regulation making it especially helpful for problems like perfectionism and anxiety that arise from a complex interaction between thoughts, feelings, and behaviors.

7.3. Acceptance and Commitment Therapy (ACT)

Instead, in ACT, mindfulness and other acceptance exercises gradually train individuals to experience their anxiety without avoidance or control. Then, building on the values exercise, individuals are taught to take concrete steps towards their values despite any unwanted private experiences, including anxiety. A new, more adaptive relationship with perfectionism can evolve from recognizing the entanglement of perfectionism with anxiety and progressing toward greater value-driven action. Exposure to one's own flaw accentuation followed by arbitrary performance tasks, thereby promoting a breakaway from the maladaptive engagement in performances that lead to feelings of anxiety. In treating perfectionism and FSAF, ACT attempts to encourage action on the basis of values and thus a breakaway from failure-avoidance (BASICS). ACT is a third wave CBT with a focus on mindfulness. It has six core concepts: cognitive defusion, self as context, present moment awareness, values, committed action, and acceptance (a hexaflex).

Another approach to managing the relationship between anxiety and perfectionism is Acceptance and Commitment Therapy (ACT), which, as a mindfulness-based approach, emphasizes psychological flexibility. Inspired by a Relational Frame Theory (RFT) of human language and cognition, ACT targets to increase the patient's ability for effective action in the service of living a vital life. ACT is unique in that the standard treatment of perfectionism helps the individual replace perfectionism with less extreme, less rigid, and more flexible standards. In ACT, the emphasis is placed not on the reduction of perfectionistic tendencies directly, rather on the reduction of the negative consequences of perfectionism (e.g., anxiety) so that commitment to action can follow naturally.

8. Self-Care Practices for Managing Anxiety and Perfectionism

Practical lifestyle changes – Increasing sleep, cutting down on alcohol, and limiting caffeine can all help to decrease levels of anxiety. Sleep deprivation can make it hard to focus, think clearly, and function effectively – and the anxiety that comes with it tends to exacerbate this, creating a vicious cycle. A good night's sleep isn't always easy to come by, and there are a variety of different ways to cultivate healthy sleep patterns, but a good first step could be trying to maintain a regular bedtime and time to wake up. For those who use it, alcohol can come with an added cause of anxiety: withdrawal. Try and offset it by drinking water and keeping hydrated.

Relaxation techniques – Meditation, mindfulness, yoga, deep breathing, and visualization are all techniques that have been proven to reduce anxiety and help practitioners feel calm. Yoga in particular focuses on the conjunction of the mind and body, and has been shown to improve mood, decrease anxiety levels, and reduce the actual physical effects of stress. There are plenty of classes and online courses that can help you learn these disciplines step by step.

Physical exercise – Keeping the body healthy helps the mind. Regular physical exercise is strongly connected with lower self-reported anxiety and higher self-esteem, and has been shown to naturally reduce anxiety pathology and symptoms. Whether it's a run, a blast at the gym, or a leisurely dog walk, exercise is a powerful tool for mental resilience. If you're feeling overwhelmed or anxious, stretching or moving your body for just five minutes can give you a moment of peaceful, focused time.

Self-care practices for managing anxiety and perfectionism

8.1. Physical Exercise and Relaxation Techniques

In the context of reducing the reciprocal influence of anxiety and perfectionism, however, found evidence that relaxation techniques, and not mindfulness, were effective. Additionally, found that worry reduction strategies, including relaxation techniques in an anxiety-perfectionism intervention, were rated very helpful or excellent by nearly half of the sample, and helpful by most of the sample. Findings suggest that relaxation techniques may be important for combating anxiety and perfectionism. These suggestions for the use of exercise and relaxation techniques in decreasing anxiety are certainly important as we work to better understand and break the anxiety-perfectionism relationship. Given that anxious perfectionists have been shown to use exercise and relaxation techniques to help manage both perfectionism and anxiety, and find these activities helpful, they may also reduce the bidirectional effects on behavior and mood.

Consistent with the well-researched effects of physical exercise on reducing anxiety, and physical exercise's influence in reducing these effects, we suggest the incorporation of exercise in anxiety-perfectionism intervention. Suggestions for the use of physical exercise for reducing anxiety are applicable when trying to reduce the reciprocal influence of anxiety and perfectionism. This includes incorporating regular physical activity that participants enjoy, which can help counteract the body's stress response. Additionally, group exercise can also be used for intervention, when social distancing or similar measures are not necessary, allowing anxious perfectionists to connect with others in healthy ways. Relaxation techniques, as well as mindfulness (an awareness practice), have been demonstrated to reduce symptoms of anxiety.

8.1.1. Anxiety

- NUTRITION: Be mindful of your nutrition. Including foods that offer a balance of complex carbohydrates, healthy fats, and protein can help reduce stress levels, support the immune system, and play a significant role in mood management. - SLEEP: Our nervous systems need rest to effectively regulate. Do your best to institute a regular sleep schedule and hygiene. - SOCIAL CONNECTIONS: Maintain connections and relationships with those around you that make you feel seen, heard, and supported. Don't have these? Seek out a new tribe that practices kindness and acceptance, such as a support group, online chat, or other communal setting. - AUDIT YOUR MEDIA DIET: What are you feeding yourself? Seek out information, entertainment, and education that supports the way you want to think.

With regard to cultivating connection and mitigating the challenges of anxiety and perfectionism, it is also helpful to think about the bigger picture and all the various interplaying aspects of wellness. The purpose of this section is to talk through a variety of habits and practices that can optimize your overall sense of well-being as we continue to engage in a deep dive of the mindsets and patterns put forth in the book "Good Moms Have Scary Thoughts." Many aspects of healthy living contribute to overall well-being, such as what we put in our bodies, what our physical environment looks like, how we move, how we process and store information, and the quality of our relationships. Delving into various mindful habits can support a decrease in the habits of anxiety and perfectionism through working with the function of our brains and nervous systems.

8.3. Journaling and Creative Outlets

Artistic Practices & Creative Outlets - Poetry, painting, drawing, and other art therapies are considered "fundamental expressive approaches." This can also include interpretive dance, music therapy, or performance. Movement, particularly dance, can be a form of embodiment therapy, using the body to release ideas, thoughts, or memories which may be so deeply repressed that even talk therapy can't reach them. These modalities can also be particularly effective with children, who may have difficulty articulating emotional states. Many times, anxiety is caused by external sources and the pressures of perfectionism. Journaling and other emotional release techniques allow for an individual to come to terms and understand these pressures, possibly helping to manage life in the future in a more proactive way.

Nurturing one's mental health through writing and self-expression can also be a tangible form of resistance to the social forces of relentless productivity. The goal of any member of an anti-capitalist movement is not to increase their productivity and value to their capitalist masters, but instead to become human and resist the inhumane seeking their annihilation. Journaling is a common form of therapy. Traditionally, a patient comes prepared with information discussed in a previous session, goals, and areas of improvement. Journaling also works as an offshoot of creative therapy. As any creative endeavor does, it opens up a side of the practitioner that might not be brought out in ordinary situations and allows them to indulge in a form of self-expression. Engaging with any creative practice, journaling included, has the potential to become a crucial emotional outlet that has many therapeutic benefits.

9. Support Systems and Community Resources for Individuals with Anxiety and Perfectionism

Social networks, Positive Peer Support, and professional guidance offer an inclusive approach, as well as a reduction in perceived social isolation. There are people in your communities, and if you are looking for them, you could get additional support. Support systems encourage seeking help, and when ready, referring someone in your networks to specialist help.

These supports come from different relationships and can provide different advantages and insights. Social networks can provide collective wisdom. Hallmark Positive Peer Support provides empathy, validation, and the reminder that you are not weird, broken, or alone. Sometimes this is just about feeling heard and understood. Our communities of care are rich with people who have "been there, done that" and might have some practical skills, problem-solving tips or techniques, or logistical assistance that could be game changers.

Being human in this world can be difficult on its hardest days, and living with anxiety and perfectionism can make the everyday challenges even harder. For many individuals, community resources and support systems can be easier to access. Based on the unique strengths and talents within these communities, creatively leveraging our collective assets could help generate some relief, support, or at the very least, help each member feel a little bit more known and cared for.

Social support, community resources, support systems, anxiety, perfectionism

10. Conclusion: Empowering Individuals to Overcome Anxiety and Perfectionism

The ultimate aim of this paper is to lay the foundations for practicing what is ultimately a personal ethos of 'good enough living', guided by the principle that 'to err is human'. It contends that allowing ourselves to be human as well as good enough is the path to reducing a potentially undoing pursuit of high standards and their untoward effects. Such a pursuit unites well-being advocacies that examine anxiety and perfectionism separately and calls for action to make their relationship better known. By doing so, we enable individuals to better recognize the potential cumulative adversities and support their psychological strategies to dismantle this feedback loop. The acknowledgement of a reciprocal anxiety-perfectionism reality encourages practitioners to take a broader, ecological approach to tackle the underlying risks associated with lifelong, and perhaps even genetic, tendencies. At its heart, this allows for the psychological interweaving of anxiety and perfectionism to be supported in a holistic approach that champions greater public insight, intervention, and support for these ubiquitous vulnerabilities.

The relationship between anxiety and perfectionism suggests that neither should be neglected when providing care and support, whether in clinical or educational contexts. Educating individuals about the circular nature of perfectionist anxiety is an important first step in breaking the cycle. By doing so, it is possible for individuals to become more aware of when they get caught in a loop of setting unrealistic goals in environments that do not provide the required resources to support such achievement. Developing such awareness could prevent these blocks from having cumulative impacts on one's life purpose and meaning. Furthermore, combining such psychoeducation with cognitive-behavioral training for reducing anxiety while building self-compassion, coping strategies, and problem-solving responses is vital, as it can give individuals the inner resources necessary to challenge and protect themselves from environmental adversity.

www.ingramcontent.com/pod-product-compliance
Lightning Source LLC
Chambersburg PA
CBHW070906260726
48661CB00004B/1622